Herbalist's Guide

to

Preventing the Flu

Janet Partlow

2014

JANET PARTLOW

ISBN:

Forthcoming books
The Herbalist's Guide to Managing Stress & Anxiety
The Herbalist's Guide to Managing Headaches
The Herbalist's Guide to Managing Menopause
The Shamanic Healer's Guide to Understanding your Empath Gift
A Naturalist's Eye: Our Life on the Water

Why a book about preventing the flu?

I have had a long interest in influenza. I was a physician assistant for thirty years and for many of those years I worked in a college health clinic. I spent far too many years working with students and watching helplessly as influenza ran unchecked through the college campus. February was a particularly hellish month where maybe 50% of the students were struggling with influenza. They were pretty motivated to avoid it, but the usual suggestions of washing hands, etc. only took us so far.

So when I began my formal herbal training in 1995 I was thrilled to learn that there are some excellent herbal remedies that can help deal with influenza.

I also have been influenced by my great-grandfather HW Partlow. He became a physician in 1885; from my elder cousins who knew him I learned that he used herbs extensively in his medical practice. In 1918 he was one of a handful of doctors working in my hometown of Olympia, Washington. When the so-called Spanish flu pandemic hit our town he was run off his feet, trying to cope with a high virulence, high fatality flu epidemic that was rampaging through the community. Usually in such pandemics, it is the health workers who die early on, but he and his family survived unscathed. That says to me that he knew his herbs and knew how to protect himself, despite his intense exposure to the virus.

Modern medicine has lost interest in herbs, but considering that viral illness are still very difficult to treat, I think we really need to be looking at other options. Hence this book.

Finally, I read an excellent book by Kathy Abascal: Herbs & Influenza: How Herbs Used in the 1918 Flu Pandemic Can Be Effective Today. She did much historical research into this pandemic and what herbs were used. I have done my own research and also utilized her suggestions to good effect. From my experience I believe we have a number of excellent plants that we can grow and keep on hand. In this book my goal is to share this information with you as we all seek to protect ourselves, our families and our communities.

Influenza or stomach flu: what do you have?

In this book I am focusing on two specific kinds of viruses. The all-purpose stomach flu is one. The other is known as influenza, which typically sweeps in waves across the United States from November through April. Here are some ways to assess what you might have.

• **Stomach flu, also known as viral gastroenteritis**: symptoms include nausea, vomiting and diarrhea. It can occur any time of year. There is rarely any fever. There are no lung symptoms such as cough, congestion or shortness of breath. While annoying and obnoxious, it is rarely serious and it rarely kills - though while you have it you may wish you were dead.

• **Influenza:** Key symptoms include: *high fever* of 100+ (in adults) for three to four days along with *aches and pains*. Sometimes the fever can be severe: 102+ in adults. (Any fever this high that persists past 24 hours means a visit to your doctor. Any persistent fever 104+ means you need to seek immediate care). Another key influenza symptom includes body aches. One viral strain that circulated in the 1890's was called "breakbone fever" because of the intense bone aches that accompanied it.

Other symptoms vary depending on the specific viral strain that is roaming in that year: you may notice a sore throat, nasal or sinus congestion, cough, or stomach symptoms such as nausea, vomiting or diarrhea. Influenza is epidemic in nature and waves of these viruses sweep through the planet each fall and winter.

Influenza can be quite debilitating while you have it. There are many types of influenza: for example H1N1 (swine flu) was a big concern a few years ago.

The influenza viruses mutate rapidly. They can also mix/ match and interchange genetic material with the flu viruses found in animals such as pigs. This makes each year's flu strain unpredictable and potentially dangerous until we see how it is playing out in human populations in that year.

A word about flu vaccines

Flu vaccines are available beginning in September of each year. Whether or not to receive one is a very personal decision. For example my spouse worked in the local school district for many years where he was exposed to swarms of kids and viruses. It made a lot of sense for him to get the vaccine and in most years, it worked well for him. For me, I don't have the same exposure risk nor do I respond well to vaccines in general, so I rely instead on herbal remedies. This has also worked well for me. So each of us needs to make up our own minds.

A word of warning: Influenza kills!

As I mentioned before, influenza virus can mutate in unpredictable and unexpected ways. Some strains develop a high virulence factor, which means that they kill at a much higher rate. For example in 1918 the Spanish flu virus emerged with a very high virulence: it had a case fatality rate of 10 - 20%, which means out of one hundred people who got it, 10 to 20 died - at least 50 million people. All around the globe, people died in droves. We need to remember this and keep alert for the arrival of such strains. Should such a strain emerge, this is one instance where I believe everyone should get a flu vaccine.

But even the usual flu kills, albeit at lower numbers. Key symptoms to watch include:

- A high fever 102+ for more than 24 hours. Or high fever 104+: seek immediate care. This is for adults. For children or elders you need to have a much higher level of concern, because the usual flu is more likely to be fatal for people in these age groups.
- If there is severe lung congestion that does not clear or if this congestion causes shortness of breath, seek immediate medical care.

- If this is an influenza that very rapidly progresses (within 24 hours) from early symptoms to serious lung congestion this suggests that the immune system is overwhelmed with a severe virus. Seek medical care immediately.

Some Herbal Precautions

In this book on herbal remedies there are several suggestions for herbs you might want to try. These herbs have not been evaluated by the Food & Drug Administration for effectiveness or safety. When you buy bottles of prepared herbs, the FDA requires this statement on the label.

In addition, herbalists are not licensed to diagnosis, treat or cure any disease.

In general it is recommended that if you have any questions about these herbal products, consult your physician.

It is also very important when it comes to flu to do self care only up to a point. Look through the section on flu symptoms to help you decide what is going on. If you have any of the danger symptoms, it is extremely important to seek immediate medical care. Most flu is benign, but occasionally, it kills. You need to keep that firmly in the front of your mind.

Once you are certain that this is the benign flu, these herbal suggestions can be very helpful. Many of us get influenza and stomach flu each year. Herbalists commonly work with people who have these viral illnesses and we tend to get excellent results.

A general rule that I follow in making herbal suggestions is that if you are taking several medications for significant health issues such as heart problems or diabetes, it is best not to blend herbs with those medications unless you have consulted with a practitioner who knows both herbs and your medications. Most modern medicine physicians are not well trained in herbal medicine. So I often refer people to naturopathic physicians who are trained in both worlds. This is the best option if you are on several medications and still want to add in herbs.

In the back of this book is a resource section. It has specific notes on how to find other healers such as herbalists, naturopaths, acupuncturists and more. Check it out!

The Viral Raid: Stopping Flu in its Tracks

Now that you have a sense of some of the symptoms, here are some ideas about the viral raid for the flu. To do this you need to have these remedies on hand.

Within first 24 hours of symptoms :

I suggest a homeopathic remedy called **Oscilliococcinium**. The name is a mouthful, but don't let that put you off: it really works. The most commonly available brand is made by Boiron and can easily be found in herb and supplement stores.

It comes in a group of three small vials of pellets. At your earliest symptoms you take one vial of pellets, then repeat every six hours until the three doses are complete.

This is a stellar influenza remedy, and is also effective for stomach flu. This is best used as a preventative in the first 24 hours of illness, where it will often stop the virus in its tracks. I have also noticed that if taken after the first twenty-four hours, it can reduce the severity and length of illness.

Homeopathics are a plant energy-based healing modality. I can't necessarily explain how they work but years of experience tells me that Oscilliococcinium is very effective. It is also safe: since there is no plant chemistry in the remedy, there is no interaction with other medications you may be taking. The trick is to have it on hand so that when the stomach flu hits at two in the morning, you have what you need.

• Black Elderberry *(Sambucus nigra or S. canadensis)* This is an herb plant that grows in Europe and eastern North America. Our ancestors from the British Isles and Ireland used it extensively in the fall and winter to prevent viral illnesses. It is believed to open up the pores to bring out heat and fluids, thus reducing a fever. It is said to open up the lungs and helps in bringing up mucous. Some recent research work in Europe found that two chemicals in elderberry can prevent the flu viruses from invading throat cells.

It is also a bitter herb, which means it helps stimulate the liver to produce more bile and to clean itself out. This is important in viral illnesses because the liver is like your own personal garbage person: it clears out the viral garbage and carts it away. You know what happens if there is a strike and household garbage starts to build up along your street? Well, the same sort of thing can occur in your body. A healthy liver that is moving out toxins & viruses means that you are less likely to get sick.

We use the berries. These are made into a syrup. A commercial preparation called Sambucol can be readily purchased in herb and supplement stores. It is also available through Amazon. (I often recommend Amazon because the price is very good and you can also read the reviews of other people who tried it.)

You can also make your own syrup and keep it in the refrigerator. In the first 24 hours of symptoms, take 1 tablespoon three times daily.

Check the back of this book for a recipe on how to make your own homemade elderberry syrup.

Precautions: if you make your own syrup, be sure to find black elderberries. In the Pacific Northwest there are red elderberries, but they can be toxic to eat. There are also blue elderberries and the jury is still out on whether these can also be toxic. The safest thing is to use only black elderberries. Check the resource page in the back of the book for places to get herbs.

You can also find or make Black Elderberry as an alcohol or glycerin based tincture. An excellent resource is Herb Pharm; their tincture products are sold across the country. Or you can make your own tincture: see recipes in the back. Take 30 drops of tincture three times daily as a viral raid.

You can also take Black Elderberry capsules. I recommend 10 - 15 capsules all at once as part of the viral raid.

Daily Prevention Against Flu Viruses

There is a season for flu viruses. Typically they start to trickle in around late September, after children have returned to school. The trickle turns into a flood by late November and is widespread by February. By May the typical flu is starting to abate as most of the human population has either had it or has become immune to it. So you want to use prevention from September through May. Here are some good choices to consider.

• Black Elderberry *(Sambucus nigra or S. canadensis)* I have talked about this herb at length in the previous section on the viral raid. You can also use it as a preventative. One tablespoon of syrup daily through the flu season should do it. Our European ancestors have used this for generations.

You can also find or make Black Elderberry as a tincture. You can buy an excellent commercial tinctures from Herb Pharm. Or you can make your own tincture: see recipes in the back. Take 30 drops of tincture daily as a preventative.

You can also take Black Elderberry capsules. I recommend 5-8 capsules a day as a preventative.

• Astragalus *(Astragalus proquinuus)*: This herb is a wonderful immune enhancer, antiviral, fever reducer, digestive tonic and adaptogen. As a preventative, it stimulates white blood cell production, increases release of antibodies, and boosts hormonal messengers that signal for virus destruction. As an adaptogen, it feeds the body's energy building apparatus over time and builds resistance to weakness and disease.

A Chinese herb in the pea family, Astragalus grows like a weed in China and can be easily grown here: it is the root that is used. As a daily herb during flu season take 5 capsules daily or 1 dropper (30 drops) of tincture daily, or stir a teaspoon of powder into a daily beverage.

• Isatis *(Isatis tinctoria)*: This herb is both antibacterial and antiviral and reduces fever. One of America's premier herbalists is Michael Tierra; he considers Isatis one of the most effective antivirals and recommends it for febrile epidemic illnesses. He considers it especially effective for infection in the lungs.

Another top herbalist, KP Khalsa, agrees with this. He feels Isatis is especially effective in a blend with Astragalas.

This is a root that is usually powdered, as it has a truly hideous bitter taste. Take five capsules a day as a preventative.

• Medicinal Mushrooms: I live in the wet side of the Pacific Northwest which is mushroom heaven. Mushrooms of many sorts erupt all around us, especially in the fall. In the last few years I became very interested in this bounty and have spent a great deal of time learning whatever I could find about them, especially the ones with medicinal qualities.

I used to think that medicinal mushrooms were like herbs in that you need a different species for different problems. When it comes to viruses, that does not appear to be true. Many kinds of these fungi are phenomenally effective at building up the immune system. So you can take them on a daily basis through the cold season and they will keep your immune system strong. One physician assistant friend of mine started doing this a few years ago and has noticed a dramatic decrease in her viral illnesses, despite the fact that she works full time in a family practice clinic, where she gets exposed to every virus on the planet.

Some mushrooms which I think are best at building up the immune system include:

• Reishi
• Turkey Tail
• Shiitake
• Cordyceps
• Agarikon

So how do you go about getting medicinal mushrooms in your body? There are a couple of excellent choices.

Paul Stamets of Fungi Perfecti has developed a great mushroom blend which he calls *Host Defense: My Community*. It has 17 different mushrooms blended together, to work synergistically to keep the immune system strong. It comes in capsule form and you take 2 capsules a day throughout the September to May cold season. Google Fungi Perfecti to find their website.

I also like to work with the people of Mushroom Harvest in Ohio. They sell bulk mushroom powders: one is a 5 mushroom blend and another is a 14 mushroom blend. You can buy anywhere from 4 ounces to a pound of these blends. You take 1-2 teaspoons a day. You can make up your own capsules (see the back of this ebook for instructions on how to do this). If you use their blend, you need 4 - 8 capsules a day.

Or you can simply stir the powder into a couple of cups of hot water, let it sit for a few minutes and drink. You can also add these powders to soups.

I like Mushroom Harvest because not only do they really know their mushrooms, but they offer them at a reasonable price. Google Mushroom Harvest to find their website.

Some non-herbal approaches to immune support

There are a number of strategies we can use to keep our immune systems healthy besides plants. From the world of the herbalist, these are some of my favorites.

• Get to bed by 11 pm each night and get the hours of sleep that your body needs. My understanding of this comes from Traditional Chinese Medicine (TCM). In that world of healing, they believe in a 24 hour body clock, whereby every two hours one organ system is at its most effective and powerful. The time from 11 pm to 3 am is the time of the gallbladder and liver. The liver plays a key role in taking out viral garbage. It turns out if you are asleep during this time you are giving the liver its best help for fighting the flu.

Some people are naturally night owls and find it hard to be asleep by 11 pm. In that case, just lie down and rest. That works almost as well.

• Limit your intake of sugar: it is documented to suppress the immune system. Since we are trying to get the immune system at its best to fight the virus, sugar is counter-productive. By sugar I mean cane sugar. Honey in small amounts is fine.

• Wash hands & cover coughs. This is the usual advice from modern medicine and it is good advice. Most virus particles enter our bodies through contact with a moist mucous membrane. Sometimes we get the virus on our hands, then rub our eyes. This is one sure-fire way to get exposed. So hand-washing is very useful.

• Manage stress: In the world of the herbalist, one of the greatest enemies I see in all my clients is stress. Stress plays a key role in knocking back the immune system. From my years as a healer, it is clear that most adults have heavy stress and some have extraordinary stress. It seems to be a chronic issue in all our lives.

We don't always have a choice about some of that stress, but we do have a choice about how we manage it. It is beyond the scope of this book to go over this topic in detail, but briefly, here are some of my favorite tools to manage stress. See if any of these speak to you:

• Some sort of meditation practice: you can find classes on Mindfulness Meditation at community centers and colleges. Yoga studios often teach meditation as well as Buddhist centers.

• Yoga: this combines breathing exercise, movement/stretching and meditation. A three for one deal! Check for local Yoga classes and studios. Community centers and community colleges often have evening classes.

• Qi Gong – This is a TCM movement practice. Acupuncturists are often required to take these classes throughout their training and afterwards, many of them teach Qi Gong. Try and find an acupuncturist in your community who can teach this. I have found this to be wonderfully relaxing. Tai Qi is a martial arts form of Qi Gong and some people prefer to do this form of movement.

• Breathing exercises. Andrew Weil has a wonderful CD called *Breathing: The Master Key to Self Healing*. It has eight exercises which can be remarkably helpful in clearing the effects of chronic stress. I especially like the 4/7/8 breath for its powerful ability to calm people down. You can google "4/7/8 Breath" on the internet and download this for free.

• Guided Imagery for Relieving Stress: Bellaruth Naperstak is a therapist who started a company called Health Journeys. She uses guided visualizations for a wide variety of health issues. Her CD on Relieving Stress is excellent and is one of my personal key tools for stress management. Google healthjourneys.com to find her website.

• Regular exercise: walking, running, swimming, or strength training, and flexibility training all can play an important role in keeping our circulatory, lymph & liver systems strong to flush out those viruses and also to clear out the biochemical effects of stress.

What if the prevention fails?

Sometimes the virus manages to sneak into our bodies, despite all our efforts to prevent it. So it is also useful to know some herbal approaches to shutting down the attack. Here are some of my favorite herbal approaches:

Early Stage Illness day 1-3: herbs to try early in the course of flu:

• Boneset (*Eupatorium perfoliatum*): This is a premier influenza herb. It is native to eastern North America and was widely used by Native tribes for influenza. The settlers also used it during bouts of what they called breakbone fever (an influenza strain that caused such bone pain it felt as if the bones would shatter). Boneset clears the aches and pains of influenza and helps the body clear out persistent fevers. It helps the liver remove the viral garbage, speeding healing. During the 1918 epidemic nearly all physicians who used herbs as their treatment modality reported that they used Boneset with great effect.

The best form of Boneset is fresh plant tincture, made from leaves and flowers; take 20-40 drops three times daily. Though it is easy to grow, by November when you need it the plant has gone back to its roots. Probably it is easiest to buy it from commercial sources such as Herb Pharm and keep on hand as needed. Or you could make fresh plant tincture in the summer and store it for future

• Agarikon (*Fomitopsis officinalis*) is a shelf mushroom or wood conk which grows out of old growth tree trunks. Historically it grew all around the world in northern wet coniferous forests. It is now almost extinct in most of the world, except in the Pacific Northwest, where Paul Stamets of Fungi Perfecti has found it and cultured it. Agarikon has been run through the Department of Defense Bio Shield program and was found to be one of the few substances with potent action against smallpox and related viruses such as swine flu, bird flu & herpes viruses. Paul has done some work with this mushroom. It has been used by Native people around the planet as a treatment for fevers, coughing, tuberculosis and asthma. In ancient Greece, Agarikon was recommended for treating respiratory illnesses, night sweats, and consumption -- later termed tuberculosis. This historical use points to some ways we can use it today. Take dried Agarikon powder: 1 teaspoon twice daily in hot water. Or try Fungi Perfecti's Host Defense Agarikon freeze dried capsules.

• Shiitake (*Lentinula edodes*) mushroom is another powerful immune system support, antiviral, and liver tonic. This is one of the few mushrooms that has undergone clinical trials in regard to its antiviral action; it turns out to be very potent. It increases natural killer cells and interferon, and fortifies the liver. In clinical trials it has decreased HIV and HSV viruses. Studies show it is very protective against virulent/lethal influenza viruses.

I suggest powdered mushroom: take 1 tsp. twice daily in tea. During a viral illness you could also make it as a mushroom soup and take daily.

• Turkey Tail (*Trametes versicolor*) is yet another mushroom that enhances the immune system, as well as being antiviral and antibacterial. It appears to assist the immune system in making natural viral killer interleukin. It also modulates immune dysfunction. This mushroom is often used in cancer treatment.

Turkey tail grows as a shelf fungus, commonly found on wet wood in our area. I recommend dried turkey tail powder, taking 5 capsules a day, or 1/2 tsp. twice daily in tea.

<u>If the flu virus continues to progress:</u>

Here are some top gun anti-influenza herbs, many of which were used in the 1918 pandemic to good effect. Since we never know when we might find ourselves in the middle of a virulent flu, I recommend that we keep tinctures of these herbs on hand. Tinctures have a long shelf life so this makes them an excellent choice for long-term storage.

• Lomatium (*lomatium dissectum*) is an herb that is an antimicrobial and antiviral with specify affinity for the respiratory system. It supports the immune system in doing its job. It helps clear the lungs of fluids. This herb is native to the Great Plains of the United States; tribal people in this area have used this plant for generations to treat lung problems, pneumonia and high fevers. During the 1918 epidemic, it was used locally to very good effect.

The root is collected and made into a tincture. Take 10-30 drops up to five times a day. It can be hard to find in nature, so your best option is to buy a commercial preparation. Herb Pharm carries it.

• Osha (*Ligusticum porteri*) is a potent antiviral and antispasmodic. It stimulates the immune system and reduces fevers, bringing on sweating which breaks fevers. Closely related to Lomatium, this plant grows at high altitude above 9500 feet (typically in the Rocky Mountains and Cascades of North America) and was used extensively by Native Americans for lung and throat infections. It is especially helpful for lung tissue, and helps the alveoli bring in more oxygen.

The root is used and either boiled in a tea or made into a tincture; 30 drops three times daily. It can also be made into an herbal honey. See the recipe section.

Herbs for specific influenza symptoms

The high virulence pandemic of 1918 killed people primarily because the lungs got overwhelmed with virus and then were flooded with fluids. People literally drowned to death. So any herbs that treat influenza need to also be effective for supporting the lungs. Here are some good choices.

• Pleurisy Root (*Asclepias tuberosa*) is an expectorant, which helps the lungs clear congestion. It is also an antispasmodic and bronchodilator, which are really important in supporting lung health during influenza. This herb was used extensively in the 1918 epidemic to help with lung involvement from the virus; it reduces inflammation and helps clear lungs and lymph.

The root is collected and dried for several months, then made into a tincture. Take 30 drops of tincture three times daily.

High virulence influenza can also cause high fever which can kill. So we look also for herbs that are helpful in reducing fever. Here are some good choices:

• Black Cohosh (*Cimicifuga racemosa*) is more commonly known as a menopause herb, but in fact was widely used by tribal people in the Appalachians as an antispasmodic, expectorant and an herb to reduce fever. This herb was used extensively in 1918, specifically for the aches, headaches and neuralgia of influenza. It was also very effective in reducing fever.

The fresh root is used to make a tincture: take 10-25 drops three times daily.

• Yarrow (*Achillea millefolium*) is a phenomenal medicinal herb with many great uses. For influenza its best use is to reduce fever. The leaves and flowers are used in a tincture: take 30 drops three times daily.

• Agarikon mushroom (*Fomitopsis officinalis*) is one I mentioned before. I think it is a great mushroom to use preventatively or in early illness, but it may also be very important in later stages. I worked with an adult who developed H1N1 (swine flu) a couple of years ago; for her it triggered her usually dormant asthma and she became very sick, very fast. We tried Agarikon and within 24 hours both the virus and her asthma were markedly reduced.

Paul Stamets of Fungi Perfecti has made a mission out of finding this mushroom and preserving many strains of it. So I would recommend getting his product Host Defense Agarikon freeze-dried capsules to keep on hand as needed.

Self care during a viral illness

During any viral illness, it is really important to take good care of ourselves. This should be obvious, but in my long years as a healer I have watched many people in the throes of an acute cold drag themselves into work because somehow they believed they were indispensable. This serves no one and ultimately just spreads the virus around to everyone else at your workplace. So let's try something novel and make a commitment to good self-care during viral illness. Here are some suggestions.

- Stay home: One of the best ways to stop a serious community flu epidemic is to impose a quarantine, where sick people rest at home and everyone else stays close to home. For healing, home is best.

- Rest is key: going to bed early, wallowing in bed for as many hours as you can, resting comfortably in a chair during the day. This is an enforced vacation: take advantage of it.

- Keep warm: viral illnesses often affect our thermostat and we can be alternately cold or hot. Keep bundled up in a comforting blankie, wear warm socks & sweats and do whatever it takes to stay warm.

- Live a low stress life, at least for a few days. Turn off the phone, ignore the doorbell, computer & cell phone. Avoid distressing news programs. Watch a favorite optimistic movie. Stare out the window and watch the birds. Watch other people race off to work & feel smug that you won't be joining the rat race that day.

- If you have stomach symptoms such as nausea, vomiting or diarrhea, give your gut a vacation from digestion. You can do a twelve hour fast from food but take small sips of fluids as you feel inclined. It is important to stay hydrated. Some good fluids might be elderberry honey tea (see recipes) Wei Qi immune support soup (see recipes). Some people use Pedialyte, which is a commercial solution for replacing electrolytes lost by vomiting or diarrhea. A simple alternative to a store-bought re-hydration solution is the following recipe from the World Health Organization:

Homemade Fluid Replacement Recipe

1 quart water

1/2 teaspoon salt

6 teaspoons sugar

You can flavor with a mild fruit juice like apple, cherry or grape. Avoid citrus juices as these can be hard on an unhappy gut.

Mix well and store in the refrigerator.

Final Word

Now you have several herbal tools to help prevent or treat stomach flu or the usual influenza. You also know when to seek medical care. Now that you have this background information, the following sections of this book will cover:

• Recipes: how to make home herbal remedies

• Resources; good books and internet resources from which you can learn more.

• Ideas about how to find a range of healers to help you with your specific health concerns. Read on!

Herbal Recipes

There are many ways to make herbal preparations and each herbalist has her/his favorites. You need to decide what works for you. In this book I'm writing down my recipes. These are simple, basic and can be easily done in your own home kitchen.

A great reference book for making herbal preparations is: The <u>Herbal Medicine Maker's Handbook</u> by James Green. This book has everything you'd ever want to know about herbal recipes and is the place I go when I am stuck.

Tinctures

Herbs are often sold in tincture form. A commercially prepared tincture has some sort of alcohol (usually pure grain alcohol); the plant material soaks in the alcohol for a while during which time the alcohol acts as a solvent and extracts all the medicine from the plant. The plant material is then strained off and you are left with the medicinal tincture.

Advantages of tinctures are these:

- They last a long time, if stored in a dark bottle in a cool dry place.
- They are easy and convenient to find in stores, and to take.
- They may be better absorbed by the body, especially if you have digestive issues.
- The medicine is very quickly available to the body.

Disadvantages that I see are:

- They are alcohol based so for people with alcoholism issues, they are not a great idea.
- They can be expensive, because you pay for not only the plants but also the alcohol solvent. For example if you want to take a month's worth of willow tincture for joint pain, the commercial cost of that tincture will run about $80.00. So it's something to consider.

- Some people really dislike the taste of the herbs in tincture, which means they may not consistently use the medicine. You need to choose a method that is most likely to be successful for you.

Here's the "folk method" for making tinctures

Get some dried plant material from the store. For the flu season you could buy some dried black elderberries. Take a clean jar with a good tight lid. Take your berries and use a food processor to grind them into powder and fill the jar 2/3 - 3/4 full of dried herb.

- Pour an alcohol solvent over it. I use potato-based vodka 100 proof, which is gluten free and cheap. Pour the vodka over the plant material nearly to the top of the jar, leaving about 1 inch space. Stir around to get the plant material well soaked. Cap off tightly with a clean lid.

- Put your jar in a sunny window, in a place where you will see it daily. Shake it down daily to stir the herbs and alcohol together. As the days progress, you will notice the alcohol is taking on the color of the plants, and the plant material is becoming brittle and lifeless.

- After 2 weeks, your tincture is done. Get another clean jar and a funnel. Line the funnel with cheesecloth and strain off your tincture. When most of the liquid seems drained off, bundle up the cheesecloth and squeeze hard, draining off the last bits.

- Cap off your jar of tincture tightly. Label and date. It's best to use a dark bottle, but the poor man's alternative is to use a mason jar and just put the tincture in a brown paper bag. Store in a cool, dark place.

If you want to make a fresh plant tincture such as boneset, collect the aerial parts (leaves & flowers and allow to wilt/dry overnight to evaporate off some of the moisture. Then chop up and proceed as you would with a dried material such as elderberries.

Powdered herbs

When I work with a client who has decided to try some herbs, we need to sort out what is the best way for him to take them. Some people are fine with tinctures: they like the ease of purchase. Other people (like me) struggle with the intense taste of some medicinal herbs, so for folks like me, powdered herbs in capsule form work best.

Advantages of powdered capsules:

- Definitely cheaper than tincture, especially if you make your own.

- You can avoid the taste of the herbs. Some herbalists consider this is a disadvantage, because the taste of the herb can have its own medicinal effects. But I tend to be practical about it: we have to find a way to get the medicine down and capsules will bypass the yuck factor.

Disadvantages of powdered capsules

- Some people have trouble swallowing capsules

- Powdered herbs tend to lose their quality quickly. I recommend using them within 6 months of purchase. There are also a lot of bad quality herb capsules being sold out there, so only buy capsules from an herb store or supplement store you trust.

- They involve more work if you go with making your own capsules.

How to make your own powdered capsules

- Get some dried plant material from the store. Or collect the material from your garden, lay out in a single layer on a window screen type of material so air can circulate. Leave in a cool, dry place until the plants are well dried. Another method is to bundle up the herbs at the base, and hang the bundle flower tips down so all the good medicine runs into the leaves and is dried there.

- Take your plant material and crumble it down. Then use a coffee mill or a food processor and grind it down to a fine powder. Some root herbs are hard to grind and may destroy your machine, so test a small amount first. One strategy with fibrous or tough roots is to freeze them for a few hours, then grind. The freezing makes them brittle and thus easier to work with. Some roots are really tough, so it's just easier to buy from the company which has already ground them down for you. (See herbal resources page.)
- The best way I have found to capsule herbs is to buy The Capsule Machine for "00" size capsules. This machine is available online or from your local herb/supplement store. You also need some size "00" capsules; I buy these online through Amazon because they are cheaper. Follow the instructions that come with the machine. These capsule machines produce 24 caps at a pop and are really slick. At our house, we sit and make capsules while we watch movies. It works well.

Herbal teas:

Let's say you want to make an herbal tea for the aches and pains of the flu. Here's a possible suggestion: Put 1 teaspoon of dried willow bark in a large cup. Pour 2 cups boiling water over the bark and let it sit for 30 minutes. Now strain out the bark and drink.

This is a medicinal tea so it will be strong. It may not taste great, but that's because you need to take enough herbs to get the effects you want. You can make it more palatable by adding honey.

Elderberry Honey Recipe

Herbal honey is a traditional way to preserve herbal medicines over time, and also a tasty way to get things down (this is especially true for picky eaters like kids). Since this was a traditional family syrup, there are many different ways to prepare these herbal honeys.

In this recipe we are making elderberry honey as a fall/winter virus preventative. It is especially useful for preventing influenza viruses. Generally the easiest way to get the berries is to buy black elderberries from a reputable herb source (see the resource list in the back of this book.

You can buy the berries whole or ground up. If they are whole, run them through an herb mill or food processor to reduce them to a powder. Then put the herbs in a double boiler pan: the bottom pan needs a few inches of water and the top pan holds the herbs. Cover the elderberries with honey to about 1 inch above the level of the herbs. Stir to make sure all the herbs are well-coated. Put a lid on the double boiler pan and bring it to a simmer. Then reduce the stove top heat to the lowest possible setting and let the herbs and honey infuse. Plan on doing this for about 4-6 hours.

Check the mixture occasionally. As you lift the lid of the pan, you will notice moisture has condensed on the lid. Use a clean towel to mop this out. Repeat several times over the hours the mixture is infusing; this process also helps remove excess moisture.

Taste the honey occasionally. When the honey picks up the taste of the herbs, you can take it off the stove. Pour the mixture through a fine mesh metal sieve to remove the herbs; pour the honey into a clean jar, put on a lid, and label and date. I store elderberry honey in the refrigerator.

Some people add other ingredients: grated fresh ginger, cloves, or cinnamon for taste.

Wei Qi immune soup

Whenever I enter the recovery phase from a flu or cold virus and my appetite starts to slowly return, I'm usually hungry for some sort of soup. In Jewish traditions, this might be a chicken soup. In China, they talk about Wei Qi soup, which is designed to strengthen the protective energetic field around us, which they call Wei Qi.

This soup can also be used preventatively. For example you might be feeling run down and everyone around you is sick: you can strengthen your Wei Qi by eating this soup.

There are many family recipes for these kinds of soups and many ingredients you could put in them. Here is my recipe:

Janet's favorite Wei Qi Soup Recipe

=1-2 tablespoons olive oil

=1 tsp fresh minced ginger

=2 carrots cut in thin rings

=2 celery ribs, cut in thin half moons

=1 -2 teaspoons of sage to taste

−1/2 teaspoon of thyme

=1 chicken breast or 2 thighs, cut into cubes (meat is optional)

Take a heavy soup pot and pour in the oil. Heat over medium heat until it shimmers, then add ginger, chicken celery and carrots. Saute until chicken has browned.

Now add 1 quart of water plus 1 quart of stock: chicken, vegetarian (I like Rapunzel's,) Mushroom stock are all good choices) You may need to add more water over the cooking time.

Now add to pot:

=1-2 medium cloves garlic, minced

=1/2 cup aduki beans

=1 cup shiitake mushrooms, sliced

(Oyster or porcini also very available and very tasty to add)

=1 burdock root: scrub and cut into rings

Simmer these veggies all together for 20 minutes until they soften.

Finish by adding in:

=1-2 bundles baby bokchoy, chopped

=4-5 green onions, sliced into rings

=2 cups shredded cabbage

=4 ounces thin rice noodles:

Simmer all these ingredients together briefly until the noodles are softened, then serve.

Optional ingredients: 1/4 cup of dried astragalus root: simmer with carrots & celery. Some people also like Miso as their stock. See what you like.

Herbal Resources

There are many places all over the world to buy herbs. I live in the Pacific Northwest and I believe it is very important to use plants that are mostly grown in my own bioregion, so I choose local herb sellers. I encourage you to do the same.

If you live someplace far away from the Northwest, I encourage you to check out your local herb stores, herbalists and supplement stores to find out about what herb sellers are available in your area. Check out your local farmer's markets: this is often a good place to find herbs.

One of my favorite strategies is to google "Herbs in__ [your town] __, USA" and see what comes up. This can help lead you to sources of herbs.

Try and find good products. Stay away from the big box stores. You can certainly buy cheap herbs at Walmart but I promise you, their primary interest is in making money. You want to spend your hard-earned money on powerful & healthy herbs that will actually give you the results you are looking for.

Places to buy herb products:

- Mountain Rose in Eugene, Oregon Use google to find them on the internet
- Herb Pharm in Williams, Oregon A great resource for tinctured herbs. Use google to find them.
- Mushroom Harvest in Athen, Ohio Use google to find them on the internet
- Fungi Perfecti near Olympia, Washington. Use google to find them on the internet.
- Western Herb Products in Gold Bar, Washington They are not on the internet, so you need to contact through their phone (360) 793-1033.

- Horizon Herbs in Williams, Oregon. This is a wonderful resource for buying living herb plants. They do a great job of shipping live plants: Use google to find them on the internet.
- You can also find live herb plants at your local farmer's market and some local nurseries.
-

My Favorite Herbal Reference Books

My first herbal teacher told us to be sure to have a big bookshelf because we would be collecting lots of herbal references. I didn't believe him. He was absolutely right; my office today has a huge shelf of books. Here is a short list of some of my favorites.

Herbal Defense, Robin Landis & KP Khalsa

Home Medicine Chest, Rosemary Gladstar

Rosemary Gladstar's Family Herbal, Rosemary Gladstar

The Holistic Herbal, David Hoffman

The Herbalist's Way, Nancy Phillips

Medicinal Plants of the Pacific West, Michael Moore

Medicinal Plants of the Mountain West, Michael Moore

The Herbal Medicine Maker's Handbook, James Green

The Way of Ayurvedic Herbs, KP Khalsa and Michael Tierra

The Way of Chinese Herbs, Michael Tierra

Herbal Therapy & Supplements, Merrily Kuhn and David Winston

The Earthwise Herbal, Matthew Wood

The Rainforest Home Remedies, Rosita Arvigo & Nadine Epstein

Healing Herbs in Ireland, Paula O'Regan

Plant Spirit Medicine 2nd Edition, Eliot Cowan

Medicinal Mushrooms, Christopher Hobbs

It takes a village: other healer resources

When we are working to improve our health, I believe that we all need a village of healers. Besides having a solid primary care physician, you may also want to consider these alternative medicine healers:

<u>Herbalists</u> There are local herbalists, some of whom are members of indigenous tribes or have other family traditions in which they have been trained. You need to ask around to find these people since some of them do not advertise. Local herb or supplement stores can often help you here.

You can also google the American Herbalist Guild. This is a professional organization that provides a certification for herbalists who choose to seek a professional credential. Look under "Our Members" and you will find a search mode for locating AHG herbalists in your area.

<u>Naturopathic Physicians</u> These are medical doctors, trained in modern medicine and also in alternative medicine. You can google the American Association of Naturopathic Physicians which has a search mode by which you can find such doctors in your community.

<u>Acupuncturists</u> Acupuncturists are formally trained and licensed in Traditional Chinese Medicine and/or Five Element Classic Chinese Medicine. You can find one in your area by asking around, or google the National Certification Commission for Acupuncture and Oriental Medicine. They have a search engine so you can find an acupuncturist in your area.

<u>Healing Touch practitioners</u> Healing Touch is an energy healing modality which works to bring the human energy field (chakras & aura) back into balance. My first training in energy medicine in 1995 was Healing Touch; I continue to use it today on myself and my clients because it is truly a profound healing modality. There are certified HT practitioners who have completed the full training (five levels). You can google Healing Touch

International and check their directory for certified practitioners in your area.

<u>Eden Energy Medicine practitioners</u> Donna Eden is a phenomenal energy medicine healer who over the last 45 years developed her own energy medicine healing tools and training program for healers. This is yet another phenomenal energy healing modality that I use on myself and clients. You can google Donna Eden at Innersource to find her state by state directory of certified Eden Energy Medicine practitioners. She also has an excellent book <u>Energy Medicine</u> 2nd edition which is full of great self-care suggestions.

My background as an herbalist

I grew up in a family of healers. My grandma was a nurse and my mom studied nursing during World War II. My great-grandfather became a doctor in 1885 in Michigan and continued his medical practice when he came to Olympia, Washington where I now live. Several of his descendants became physicians. There was a certain pressure on me to become a doctor but somehow the pressure never quite took. I ended up finishing my college degree by becoming a physician assistant (PA) with a specialty in women's health care. I later went back to the University of Washington where I got additional training in Medex NW, becoming a PA in family medicine in 1980. I took an early retirement from that work in 2002.

Around 1995 the medicine of plants began to call to me. I had developed rheumatoid arthritis and despite the efforts of an excellent rheumatologist, nothing she did nor prescribed offered any relief. I was also working in a college health center; many of my young adult patients were very interested in herbal medicine and were disappointed that I had no training and expertise to offer in this area. I was desperate to find relief from my arthritis pain and also under pressure from my patients, so I began my studies in herbal medicine.

It was one of the best choices I ever made in my life. The world of plants has opened me up to a profound world of healing And it was only a little while ago I learned from one of my older cousins, a grandson of Dr. H. W. Partlow, that our ancestor HW had two offices in Olympia's Security Building: one was his treatment room and the other was stuffed full of HW's favorite healing herbs.

So it all comes around, full circle.

My formal herbal training

Clinical Herbalist Certification Program. KP Khalsa, 1998-1999

Clinical Herbalist Apprenticeship. KP Khalsa, 1999

Certification Course in Aromatherapy. Kurt Schnaubelt, 2000

East-West Herb Course. Michael & Leslie Tierra, 2001

Therapeutic Herbalism Course. David Hoffman, 2002

Spirit of the Plants (Plant Spirit Medicine) Joyce Netishen, 2001-02

Foundations in Herbal Medicine. Dr. Tierona LowDog, 2002

Pacific School of Herbal Medicine. Adam Seller, 2002

The Science & Art of Herbalism. Rosemary Gladstar, 2004

School of Traditional Hispanic Herbalism. Charles Garcia, 2005

I became a professional member of the American Herbalist Guild in 2001.

Other formal plant & botany studies:

Botany 112, South Puget Sound Community College,
        Laine McLaughlin, 2002

Wetland Plants of the Northwest,
        University of Washington, Sarah Cooke, 2004

Other important teachers, many of whom I know from their books:

Michael Moore, Medicinal Plants of the Pacific West

Christopher Hobbs, Medicinal Mushrooms

Nancy Phillips, The Herbalist's Way

David Winston, Adaptogens

Matthew Woods, The Earthwise Herbal

Rosita Arvigo, Rainforest Remedies

Juliette de Bairacli Levy, (Juliette of the Herbs, film by Tish Streeten)

I owe a special thanks to two of my earliest herbal teachers: Elise Krohn and Joyce Netishen, who have walked the beauty way of plants as long as I have known them and have been very generous in sharing their knowledge with me and others. I am very grateful to have had the opportunity to walk alongside them.

Other important herbalist/acupuncturist friends include Rain Delvin and Susan Monaco, superb healers and wonderful teachers for me along my path.

www.ingramcontent.com/pod-product-compliance
Lightning Source LLC
Chambersburg PA
CBHW070242290526
45789CB00004B/1730

* 9 7 8 1 5 0 2 3 7 3 5 6 4 *